FIT IN A FLASH: 30-MINUTE WORKOUTS FOR BUSY LIVES

Efficient Workouts for a Busy Lifestyle

TABLE OF CONTENT

Part 2: 30-Minute Workout Plans

Part 3: Specialized Workouts

Welcome to Fit in a Flash

In today's fast-paced world, finding time for fitness can feel like an impossible challenge. Juggling work, family, and social commitments often leaves little room for lengthy gym sessions or elaborate workout routines. That's where "Fit in a Flash: 30-Minute Workouts for Busy Lives" comes in. This book is designed to provide you with quick, effective, and manageable workouts that fit seamlessly into your busy schedule, helping you achieve and maintain fitness without sacrificing other important aspects of your life.

The Importance of Fitness in a Busy World

Maintaining physical fitness is crucial for overall health and well-being, yet it's often one of the first things to be neglected when life gets hectic. Regular exercise is not just about maintaining a certain physique; it's about improving mental health, boosting energy levels, and enhancing your quality of life. Even with a packed schedule, incorporating short, high-impact workouts can make a significant difference.

With increasing demands on our time, it's more important than ever to find efficient ways to stay active. Exercise can reduce stress, improve sleep, and increase productivity, making it an essential component of a balanced, healthy lifestyle. "Fit in a Flash" offers a practical solution for anyone looking to integrate fitness into their daily routine without compromising on time.

How to Use This Book

"Fit in a Flash: 30-Minute Workouts for Busy Lives" is structured to help you quickly and easily find the right workouts for your needs and schedule. Here's how to make the most of it:

1. **Identify Your Goals**: Whether you want to lose weight, build muscle, increase flexibility, or simply stay active, start by identifying your fitness goals. This will help you choose the workouts that are most effective for you.

2. **Choose Your Workout**: The book is divided into sections based on workout types and fitness levels. Whether you have a full 30 minutes or only a fraction of that, you'll find routines tailored to your available time and desired intensity.

3. **Follow the Plan**: Each workout plan is designed to be straightforward and easy to follow. Detailed instructions and tips are provided to ensure you perform exercises safely and effectively.

4. **Stay Consistent**: Consistency is key to seeing results. Use the suggested weekly schedules to keep your workouts varied and interesting, preventing burnout and keeping you motivated.

5. **Adapt and Adjust**: As you progress, feel free to adapt the workouts to suit your evolving fitness level. The flexibility of the routines allows for adjustments, ensuring they remain challenging and rewarding.

By integrating these quick, high-impact workouts into your daily routine, you'll discover that maintaining fitness is not only possible but also enjoyable and rewarding. Welcome to "Fit in a Flash"—your guide to staying fit, healthy, and energized in a busy world. Let's get started!

PART 1: GETTING STARTED

CHAPTER 1: UNDERSTANDING FITNESS FUNDAMENTALS

The Science of Effective Workouts

In the world of fitness, not all workouts are created equal. Understanding the science behind effective exercise can help you make the most out of every minute you invest in your health. Our bodies respond to physical stress in specific ways, and by leveraging this knowledge, you can achieve maximum results with minimal time.

Effective workouts are those that engage multiple muscle groups, elevate your heart rate, and challenge your body in new ways. This combination triggers various physiological responses: increased calorie burn, improved cardiovascular health, and enhanced muscle strength and endurance. High-intensity workouts, even in short bursts, stimulate the production of hormones like adrenaline and growth hormone, which play critical roles in fat burning and muscle growth.

The key to an effective workout lies in its intensity and variety. By incorporating elements such as strength training, cardiovascular exercise, and flexibility, you create a well-rounded fitness routine that promotes overall health. This approach not only helps you achieve specific fitness goals faster but also keeps your routine interesting and sustainable.

Benefits of Short, Intense Workouts

In our fast-paced lives, time is a precious commodity. Thankfully, you don't need hours at the gym to see significant health benefits. Short, intense workouts, such as those featured in "Fit in a Flash," offer numerous advantages that align perfectly with a busy lifestyle.

1. **Time Efficiency**: One of the most obvious benefits is the time saved. A 30-minute workout can fit into the busiest of schedules, making it easier to stay consistent. This consistency is crucial for long-term success and overall health improvement.

2. **Increased Metabolism**: High-intensity workouts elevate your heart rate and keep it high throughout the session. This boost continues even after the workout is done, thanks to the afterburn effect (excess post-exercise oxygen consumption or EPOC). This means your body continues to burn calories at an increased rate for hours after you've finished exercising.

3. **Enhanced Cardiovascular Health**: Short, intense sessions are excellent for improving heart health. They help lower blood pressure, increase circulation, and reduce the risk of cardiovascular diseases by strengthening the heart and improving its efficiency.

4. **Muscle Growth and Fat Loss**: High-intensity workouts often combine strength and cardio, which are essential for building lean muscle and burning fat. This combination helps sculpt a toned physique while shedding unwanted pounds.

5. **Improved Mental Health**: Exercise releases endorphins, the body's natural mood lifters. Even a short workout can significantly reduce stress, anxiety, and depression, leaving you feeling more energized and focused.

6. **Flexibility and Adaptability**: The beauty of short, intense workouts is their versatility. They can be done

<u>anywhere, with minimal or no equipment, making them perfect for home, office, or travel.</u>

By incorporating these powerful, science-backed workouts into your daily routine, you can achieve a higher level of fitness without sacrificing time. The journey to a healthier, fitter you doesn't have to be a long one—just a consistent, intentional one. Embrace the power of short, intense workouts and experience the transformative benefits they bring to your life. Welcome to the beginning of your "Fit in a Flash" journey!

CHAPTER 2: PREPARING FOR SUCCESS

Setting Realistic Goals

Embarking on a fitness journey is an exciting and transformative endeavor, but setting realistic goals is crucial to sustaining motivation and achieving long-term success. Unrealistic expectations can lead to frustration and burnout, while attainable goals keep you focused and encouraged.

Start by defining what you want to achieve. Are you looking to lose weight, build muscle, improve your cardiovascular health, or simply feel more energetic? Be specific. For example, instead of aiming to "get fit," set a goal to "lose 10 pounds in three months" or "run a 5K in six weeks." Specific goals provide a clear target and a roadmap for your efforts.

Break down your larger goal into smaller, manageable milestones. Celebrate each victory, no matter how small, as this builds momentum and confidence. Remember, fitness is a marathon, not a sprint. Consistent progress, no matter how incremental, leads to significant changes over time.

Essential Equipment and Space

One of the advantages of "Fit in a Flash: 30-Minute Workouts for Busy Lives" is the minimal equipment required. You don't need a fully stocked gym to achieve great results. However, having a few essential items can enhance your workout experience and effectiveness.

Basic Equipment:

- **Resistance Bands**: Versatile and portable, they provide resistance for strength training and can be easily adjusted for different exercises.

- **Dumbbells**: A pair of light to medium weights (5-15 pounds) can add intensity to your workouts.

- **Yoga Mat**: Provides a comfortable surface for floor exercises and stretching.

- **Jump Rope**: An excellent tool for quick cardio sessions.

- **Water Bottle**: Staying hydrated is crucial during any workout.

Creating Your Space: Designate a small area in your home or office for your workouts. It doesn't need to be large, but it should be free from distractions and have enough room for you to move comfortably. Clear away any clutter and ensure you have proper ventilation and lighting. This dedicated space will help you stay focused and make your workout time more enjoyable.

Assessing Your Fitness Level

Before diving into your new fitness routine, it's important to assess your current fitness level. This will help you choose the right workouts and track your progress effectively.

Self-Assessment:

- **Cardiovascular Endurance**: Test your endurance by timing how long you can maintain a steady pace while jogging or using a stationary bike. Note your heart rate and how quickly it returns to normal after stopping.

- **Strength**: Perform basic exercises like push-ups, squats, and planks to gauge your current strength level. Count the number of repetitions or the duration you can hold a plank to set a baseline.

- **Flexibility**: Assess your flexibility with stretches like the seated forward bend or shoulder stretch. Note how far you can reach or how comfortable you feel during these

<u>stretches.</u>

Professional Assessment:

- <u>Consider consulting a fitness professional or personal trainer for a more detailed evaluation. They can provide personalized insights and help tailor your workouts to your specific needs and goals.</u>

Regularly reassessing your fitness level as you progress is essential. It allows you to adjust your workouts to keep them challenging and ensures you're moving towards your goals. Remember, fitness is a journey, and understanding where you start is the first step to getting where you want to be.

By setting realistic goals, equipping yourself with the basics, and understanding your starting point, you're laying a solid foundation for success. Let's get ready to transform your fitness routine with "Fit in a Flash" and make every minute count!

CHAPTER 3: CREATING A SUSTAINABLE ROUTINE

Time Management Tips for Busy Schedules

Incorporating fitness into a hectic lifestyle may seem daunting, but with the right time management strategies, it's entirely achievable. The key is to maximize the efficiency of your workouts and seamlessly integrate them into your daily routine.

1. Prioritize Your Health:

- Treat your workouts like important meetings or appointments. Schedule them into your calendar and stick to them. Consistency is crucial for long-term success.

2. Utilize Micro Workouts:

- Short bursts of exercise can be just as effective as longer sessions. Fit in quick workouts during breaks, such as a 10-minute HIIT session before breakfast or a fast-paced walk during lunch.

3. Combine Activities:

- Multitask where possible. Turn household chores into a workout, or do calf raises while brushing your teeth. These small additions can add up over time.

4. Plan Ahead:

- Prepare your workout clothes and equipment the

night before. Having everything ready to go minimizes excuses and helps you stay committed.

5. Set a Routine:

- Establish a consistent time for your workouts, whether it's first thing in the morning, during a lunch break, or in the evening. A regular schedule helps form a habit.

Overcoming Common Barriers

Even with the best intentions, life can throw obstacles in your path. Here's how to overcome some common barriers to maintaining a fitness routine.

1. Lack of Time:

- **Solution:** Prioritize short, high-intensity workouts. "Fit in a Flash" offers 30-minute routines that deliver maximum results in minimal time. Remember, some exercise is better than none. Consistency, even in short durations, is key.

2. Low Motivation:

- **Solution:** Set specific, achievable goals and track your progress. Celebrate small victories to stay motivated. Joining a fitness group or finding a workout buddy can also provide accountability and encouragement.

3. Boredom:

- **Solution:** Variety is the spice of life. Mix up your workouts to keep them exciting. Alternate between cardio, strength training, and flexibility exercises to stay engaged and challenged. "Fit in a Flash" provides a diverse range of routines to keep you interested.

4. Limited Space or Equipment:

- **Solution:** Utilize bodyweight exercises that require minimal space and no equipment. Exercises like push-ups, squats, and planks can be done anywhere. Resistance bands and dumbbells are also great, compact options that enhance your workouts without taking up much room.

5. Fatigue and Stress:

- **Solution:** Listen to your body. If you're feeling exhausted, opt for a gentle workout or stretching session instead of an intense one. Exercise can actually boost your energy levels and reduce stress, so finding the right balance is crucial.

By addressing these common barriers and implementing effective time management strategies, you can create a sustainable fitness routine that fits seamlessly into your busy life. Remember, the goal is to make fitness a regular part of your routine, not an additional source of stress.

Building on the foundation of setting realistic goals and preparing your space from Chapter 2, you're now equipped to create a routine that not only fits into your life but enhances it. Embrace the journey with "Fit in a Flash" and discover how small, consistent efforts can lead to significant, lasting changes in your health and well-being.

PART 2: 30-MINUTE WORKOUT PLANS

CHAPTER 4: QUICK CARDIO BLASTS

Welcome to the heart-pumping world of quick cardio blasts! In this chapter, we dive into two powerful and efficient forms of cardiovascular exercise designed to maximize your fitness results in just 30 minutes: High-Intensity Interval Training (HIIT) and Tabata Workouts. These routines are perfect for busy lives, helping you burn calories, boost metabolism, and improve cardiovascular health in a fraction of the time.

High-Intensity Interval Training (HIIT)

High-Intensity Interval Training, or HIIT, is a workout strategy that alternates between short bursts of intense exercise and brief periods of rest or lower-intensity exercise. This approach pushes your body to its limits, leading to increased calorie burn and improved fitness levels in less time.

Benefits of HIIT:

- **Efficient Calorie Burn:** HIIT workouts keep your heart rate up, burning more fat in less time. The afterburn effect (EPOC) means you'll continue to burn calories even after the workout is over.

- **Improved Cardiovascular Health:** HIIT improves heart health by challenging your cardiovascular system with high-intensity intervals.

- **Adaptability:** HIIT can be adapted to any fitness level and requires little to no equipment. You can perform HIIT with bodyweight exercises, running, cycling, or any other form of cardio.

Sample HIIT Routine:

1. **Warm-Up:** 5 minutes of light jogging or dynamic stretching.
2. **Work Interval:** 30 seconds of high-intensity exercise (e.g., sprinting, jumping jacks, burpees).
3. **Rest Interval:** 30 seconds of low-intensity exercise or rest.
4. **Repeat:** Alternate between work and rest intervals for 20 minutes.
5. **Cool Down:** 5 minutes of walking or stretching to bring your heart rate down gradually.

HIIT Tips:

- Start with a ratio that suits your fitness level, such as 20 seconds of work and 40 seconds of rest.
- As you improve, increase the duration of the high-intensity intervals and decrease the rest periods.
- Mix up exercises to keep your workouts engaging and to challenge different muscle groups.

Tabata Workouts

Tabata is a specific type of HIIT that follows a precise 20-seconds-on, 10-seconds-off format for a total of 4 minutes per exercise. This protocol, developed by Japanese scientist Dr. Izumi Tabata, is known for its efficiency and effectiveness.

Benefits of Tabata:

- **Time-Saving:** Each Tabata workout consists of just 4 minutes of high-intensity effort, making it perfect for those with tight schedules.
- **High Caloric Burn:** Despite its short duration, Tabata can burn significant calories due to its intense nature.
- **Versatility:** Tabata can be performed with a variety of exercises, from bodyweight moves to kettlebell swings.

Sample Tabata Routine:

1. **Warm-Up:** 5 minutes of light cardio or dynamic stretching.

2. **Exercise 1:** 20 seconds of high-intensity exercise (e.g., squat jumps), followed by 10 seconds of rest. Repeat 8 times.

3. **Exercise 2:** 20 seconds of a different high-intensity exercise (e.g., push-ups), followed by 10 seconds of rest. Repeat 8 times.

4. **Continue:** Perform additional Tabata sets with different exercises if desired, up to a total of 30 minutes.

5. **Cool Down:** 5 minutes of light activity or stretching.

Tabata Tips:

- Focus on maintaining proper form during the high-intensity intervals to prevent injury.

- Choose exercises that engage multiple muscle groups for a full-body workout.

- Use a timer or Tabata app to keep track of intervals and stay on pace.

Incorporating HIIT and Tabata workouts into your fitness routine is a game-changer, especially for those with busy lives. These quick cardio blasts offer maximum results in minimal time, aligning perfectly with the sustainable routines we discussed in Chapter 3. By making the most of every minute, you'll be well on your way to achieving your fitness goals with "Fit in a Flash: 30-Minute Workouts for Busy Lives."

Let's get your heart racing and your body moving with these exhilarating, efficient cardio workouts!

CHAPTER 5: STRENGTH IN MINUTES

Welcome to "Strength in Minutes," where we harness the power of efficient, time-saving workouts to build and tone your muscles. Strength training is an essential component of a well-rounded fitness routine, and with our 30-minute plans, you can achieve impressive results without spending hours in the gym. Building on the quick cardio blasts from Chapter 4, these strength workouts complement your cardio efforts by enhancing muscle definition and overall strength.

Full-Body Strength Circuits

Full-body strength circuits are designed to target multiple muscle groups in one session, providing a balanced workout that boosts metabolism and builds lean muscle. These circuits keep your heart rate up, combining the benefits of strength training and cardio for an effective calorie burn.

Benefits of Full-Body Strength Circuits:

- **Comprehensive Conditioning**: Engage all major muscle groups for a complete workout.
- **Time Efficiency:** Maximize your workout time with exercises that hit multiple areas simultaneously.
- **Variety:** Keep workouts interesting and prevent plateaus by constantly challenging different muscles.

Sample Full-Body Strength Circuit:

1. **Warm-Up:** 5 minutes of dynamic stretches or light cardio.
2. **Circuit:**
   - **Squats**: 12 reps
   - **Push-Ups**: 12 reps
   - **Bent-Over Rows**: 12 reps
   - **Lunges**: 12 reps per leg
   - **Plank**: Hold for 30 seconds
3. **Repeat:** Perform the circuit 3 times with minimal rest between exercises.
4. **Cool Down:** 5 minutes of stretching to enhance flexibility and recovery.

Full-Body Tips:

- Focus on form and controlled movements to maximize effectiveness and reduce injury risk.
- Adjust weights and repetitions based on your fitness level and progression.

Upper Body Focus

An upper body workout zeroes in on the muscles of the chest, back, shoulders, and arms. Strengthening these areas not only improves aesthetics but also enhances functional fitness, making daily tasks easier.

Benefits of Upper Body Workouts:

- **Enhanced Definition:** Build and tone muscles for a sculpted upper body.
- **Functional Strength:** Improve your ability to perform everyday tasks, such as lifting and carrying.
- **Posture Improvement:** Strengthen the back and shoulders to support better posture.

Sample Upper Body Workout:

1. **Warm-Up:** 5 minutes of arm circles and light cardio.

2. **Workout:**
   - **Chest Press**: 12 reps
   - **Dumbbell Rows**: 12 reps per side
   - **Shoulder Press**: 12 reps
   - **Bicep Curls**: 15 reps
   - **Tricep Dips**: 15 reps

3. **Repeat:** Complete the circuit 3 times, resting as needed between sets.

4. **Cool Down:** 5 minutes of stretching, focusing on the upper body muscles.

Upper Body Tips:

- Use weights that challenge you but allow for proper form throughout the exercises.
- Incorporate a variety of movements to engage different parts of the upper body.

Lower Body Focus

Focusing on the lower body targets the legs, glutes, and hips. These exercises build strength and power, enhance balance, and improve overall athletic performance.

Benefits of Lower Body Workouts:

- **Increased Strength:** Develop powerful legs and glutes, essential for everyday movements.
- **Improved Balance:** Strengthen stabilizing muscles to enhance balance and prevent falls.
- **Boosted Calorie Burn:** Large lower body muscles burn more calories, aiding in weight management.

Sample Lower Body Workout:

1. **Warm-Up:** 5 minutes of leg swings and light cardio.
2. **Workout:**
   - **Squats**: 15 reps
   - **Deadlifts**: 12 reps

- **Lunges**: 12 reps per leg
- **Glute Bridges**: 15 reps
- **Calf Raises**: 20 reps

3. **Repeat:** Perform the circuit 3 times with minimal rest between exercises.

4. **Cool Down:** 5 minutes of stretching, focusing on the lower body muscles.

Lower Body Tips:

- Prioritize proper form, especially with exercises like squats and deadlifts, to prevent injury.
- Gradually increase weight and intensity as your strength improves.

By incorporating these targeted strength circuits into your routine, you'll not only build and tone muscle but also enhance your overall fitness and performance. These workouts are designed to complement the cardio blasts from Chapter 4, providing a comprehensive fitness plan that fits seamlessly into your busy life.

Get ready to feel stronger, more confident, and energized with "Fit in a Flash: 30-Minute Workouts for Busy Lives." Let's build that strength in minutes and transform your body efficiently and effectively!

CHAPTER 6: CORE POWER

Welcome to "Core Power," where we focus on building a strong, stable, and sculpted core. A powerful core is essential for overall fitness, improving posture, enhancing balance, and supporting all other movements. Following the strength routines from Chapter 5, these 30-minute core workouts will help you develop a solid foundation that complements your full-body and targeted strength exercises.

Abdominal and Core Strength Workouts

A well-defined core isn't just about aesthetics; it's about functional strength that supports your entire body. These workouts target the abdominal muscles, obliques, lower back, and hips, providing a comprehensive approach to core conditioning.

Benefits of Abdominal and Core Strength Workouts:

- **Improved Stability:** A strong core enhances balance and stability, reducing the risk of falls and injuries.

- **Better Posture:** Strengthening your core helps maintain proper posture, reducing strain on your spine and alleviating back pain.

- **Enhanced Performance:** A solid core supports all physical activities, from daily tasks to athletic endeavors.

Sample Abdominal and Core Workout:

1. **Warm-Up:** 5 minutes of light cardio and dynamic stretches, focusing on the torso.

2. **Workout:**
   - **Plank**: Hold for 60 seconds
   - **Bicycle Crunches**: 20 reps per side
   - **Russian Twists**: 20 reps per side
   - **Leg Raises**: 15 reps
   - **Mountain Climbers**: 20 reps per side

3. **Repeat:** Perform the circuit 3 times with minimal rest between exercises.

4. **Cool Down:** 5 minutes of stretching, focusing on the abdominal muscles and lower back.

Core Workout Tips:

- Maintain proper form to maximize effectiveness and prevent injury. Engage your core throughout each exercise.

- Progress by increasing the duration or intensity of the exercises as your strength improves.

Pilates-Inspired Core Sessions

Pilates is renowned for its focus on core strength, flexibility, and mindful movement. These Pilates-inspired sessions incorporate controlled, precise exercises that build deep core strength and improve overall body awareness.

Benefits of Pilates-Inspired Core Sessions:

- **Mind-Body Connection:** Enhance your awareness of movement and improve coordination.

- **Increased Flexibility:** Pilates exercises promote flexibility, especially in the spine and hips.

- **Low Impact:** These sessions are gentle on the joints, making them suitable for all fitness levels.

Sample Pilates-Inspired Core Workout:

1. **Warm-Up:** 5 minutes of gentle stretching and deep breathing.

2. **Workout:**
   - **Hundred**: 100 pulses with controlled breathing
   - **Roll-Up**: 10 reps
   - **Single Leg Stretch**: 15 reps per leg
   - **Double Leg Stretch**: 15 reps
   - **Criss-Cross**: 20 reps per side

3. **Repeat:** Perform the circuit 3 times with controlled movements and focus on form.

4. **Cool Down:** 5 minutes of gentle stretching, focusing on the core and spine.

Pilates Tips:

- Focus on controlled, deliberate movements. Quality over quantity is key in Pilates.
- Use your breath to enhance the exercises, inhaling to prepare and exhaling to execute the movement.

By integrating these core power workouts into your routine, you'll not only achieve a toned midsection but also build the foundational strength needed for overall fitness and stability. These routines are the perfect complement to the full-body and targeted strength workouts from Chapter 5, ensuring a balanced and comprehensive approach to your fitness journey.

With "Fit in a Flash: 30-Minute Workouts for Busy Lives," you can develop a strong, resilient core that supports all your activities and enhances your quality of life. Let's harness the power of your core and take your fitness to the next level!

CHAPTER 7: FLEXIBILITY AND MOBILITY

Welcome to "Flexibility and Mobility," a vital component of the "Fit in a Flash" program that enhances your overall fitness by improving your range of motion and preventing injuries. Flexibility and mobility exercises are the perfect complement to the strength and core workouts from Chapter 6, ensuring your body remains agile and resilient. In this chapter, we'll explore Quick Yoga Flows and Dynamic Stretching Routines designed to fit seamlessly into your busy schedule.

Quick Yoga Flows

Yoga is a fantastic way to improve flexibility, reduce stress, and promote overall well-being. Quick yoga flows are designed to fit into your 30-minute workout plan, providing a rejuvenating break that enhances your physical and mental health.

Benefits of Quick Yoga Flows:

- **Increased Flexibility:** Regular practice helps lengthen and stretch muscles, improving flexibility over time.
- **Stress Reduction:** Yoga encourages mindfulness and deep breathing, reducing stress and promoting relaxation.
- **Enhanced Recovery:** Gentle yoga flows aid in muscle recovery and prevent soreness after intense workouts.

Sample Quick Yoga Flow:

1. **Warm-Up:** 5 minutes of deep breathing and gentle stretches.
2. **Flow:**
   - **Cat-Cow Pose**: 1 minute
   - **Downward-Facing Dog**: 1 minute
   - **Warrior I**: 1 minute per side
   - **Warrior II**: 1 minute per side
   - **Triangle Pose**: 1 minute per side
   - **Seated Forward Bend**: 2 minutes
   - **Child's Pose**: 2 minutes
3. **Repeat:** Perform the sequence 2 times, focusing on smooth transitions and deep breathing.
4. **Cool Down:** 5 minutes of deep relaxation in Corpse Pose (Savasana).

Yoga Flow Tips:

- Focus on your breath, inhaling and exhaling deeply to enhance each stretch and pose.
- Move slowly and mindfully, paying attention to how your body feels in each position.

Dynamic Stretching Routines

Dynamic stretching involves active movements that stretch your muscles and improve your range of motion. These routines are perfect for warming up before a workout or as a stand-alone session to boost flexibility and mobility.

Benefits of Dynamic Stretching:

- **Improved Range of Motion:** Dynamic stretches help increase your range of motion, making movements easier and more fluid.
- **Injury Prevention:** Warming up your muscles with dynamic stretches reduces the risk of injuries during workouts.

- **Enhanced Performance:** Preparing your muscles and joints for activity improves overall performance in physical activities.

Sample Dynamic Stretching Routine:

1. **Warm-Up:** 5 minutes of light cardio, such as jogging or jumping jacks.
2. **Routine:**
   - **Leg Swings**: 1 minute per leg
   - **Arm Circles**: 1 minute each direction
   - **Lunge with Twist**: 1 minute per side
   - **High Knees**: 1 minute
   - **Torso Rotations**: 1 minute
   - **Butt Kicks**: 1 minute
   - **Hip Circles**: 1 minute each direction
3. **Repeat:** Perform the sequence 2 times, keeping movements controlled and deliberate.
4. **Cool Down:** 5 minutes of static stretching, focusing on major muscle groups.

Dynamic Stretching Tips:

- Keep movements controlled and avoid bouncing or jerky motions to prevent injury.
- Incorporate dynamic stretches into your warm-up to prepare your body for more intense activity.

By integrating these flexibility and mobility exercises into your fitness routine, you'll enhance your body's ability to perform and recover. These routines work hand-in-hand with the core strengthening from Chapter 6, ensuring a well-rounded approach to your health and fitness.

With "Fit in a Flash: 30-Minute Workouts for Busy Lives," you can enjoy the benefits of increased flexibility and mobility, making every aspect of your fitness journey more enjoyable and effective. Let's stretch, flow, and move with ease, enhancing your overall wellness and keeping your body ready for any challenge!

CHAPTER 8: COMBINING WORKOUTS

Welcome to "Combining Workouts," where we bring together the best of cardio, strength, and flexibility to create balanced and effective fitness routines. This chapter will guide you on how to mix cardio and strength exercises for maximum impact and outline balanced weekly schedules to ensure you get the most out of your 30-minute workouts. Building on the flexibility and mobility practices from Chapter 7, these combined workouts will help you achieve a well-rounded fitness regimen that fits seamlessly into your busy life.

Mixing Cardio and Strength

Combining cardio and strength exercises in a single workout can elevate your fitness routine to a new level. This approach maximizes calorie burn, builds muscle, and improves cardiovascular health, all within the same session.

Benefits of Mixing Cardio and Strength:

- **Time Efficiency:** Get the benefits of both cardio and strength training in one session, saving time while still achieving your fitness goals.

- **Enhanced Results:** Combining these elements boosts metabolism, increases muscle tone, and improves endurance.

- **Variety:** Mixing different types of exercises keeps your

<u>workouts interesting and engaging.</u>

Sample Combined Workout:

1. **Warm-Up:** 5 minutes of dynamic stretching or light cardio.

2. **Workout:**
   - **Circuit 1:**
     - **Jumping Jacks:** 1 minute
     - **Push-Ups:** 15 reps
     - **High Knees:** 1 minute
     - **Squats:** 15 reps
   - **Circuit 2:**
     - **Burpees:** 1 minute
     - **Dumbbell Rows:** 15 reps per side
     - **Mountain Climbers:** 1 minute
     - **Lunges:** 15 reps per leg

3. **Repeat:** Perform each circuit 2 times with minimal rest between exercises.

4. **Cool Down:** 5 minutes of static stretching, focusing on the muscles used.

Combining Tips:

- Alternate between cardio and strength exercises to keep your heart rate up and muscles engaged.
- Choose compound movements that work multiple muscle groups for maximum efficiency.

Balanced Weekly Schedules

Creating a balanced weekly schedule ensures you're targeting all aspects of fitness: strength, cardio, flexibility, and rest. A well-rounded plan prevents overtraining, reduces injury risk, and helps you stay motivated.

Benefits of a Balanced Weekly Schedule:

- **Comprehensive Fitness:** Address all areas of fitness to improve overall health and performance.

- **Injury Prevention:** Balance intense workouts with rest and recovery to prevent burnout and injuries.
- **Consistent Progress:** Regular, varied workouts help you progress steadily and avoid plateaus.

Sample Weekly Schedule:

- **Monday:**
    - **Workout:** Full-Body Strength Circuit (Chapter 5)
    - **Focus:** Building muscle and strength
- **Tuesday:**
    - **Workout:** Quick Cardio Blast (Chapter 4)
    - **Focus:** Improving cardiovascular health and endurance
- **Wednesday:**
    - **Workout:** Core Power (Chapter 6)
    - **Focus:** Strengthening the core and improving stability
- **Thursday:**
    - **Workout:** Flexibility and Mobility (Chapter 7)
    - **Focus:** Enhancing flexibility and promoting recovery
- **Friday:**
    - **Workout:** Upper Body Focus (Chapter 5)
    - **Focus:** Targeting and toning upper body muscles
- **Saturday:**
    - **Workout:** Lower Body Focus (Chapter 5)
    - **Focus:** Strengthening and sculpting the lower body
- **Sunday:**
    - **Workout:** Rest or Gentle Yoga Flow (Chapter 7)
    - **Focus:** Rest and recovery

Scheduling Tips:

- Listen to your body and adjust the schedule as needed to match your fitness level and recovery needs.

- Include a mix of high-intensity and lower-intensity workouts to maintain balance and prevent overtraining.

- Stay flexible with your routine. If you miss a workout, don't stress—just pick up where you left off.

By combining different types of workouts and following a balanced weekly schedule, you'll maximize your results and maintain a sustainable fitness routine. These strategies complement the flexibility and mobility routines from Chapter 7, ensuring you stay agile and ready for any physical challenge.

With "Fit in a Flash: 30-Minute Workouts for Busy Lives," you can create an effective, enjoyable, and sustainable fitness plan that fits perfectly into your busy lifestyle. Let's blend cardio, strength, and flexibility to achieve your ultimate fitness goals and enjoy the journey to a healthier, stronger you!

PART 3: SPECIALIZED WORKOUTS

CHAPTER 9: WORKOUTS FOR BEGINNERS

Welcome to "Workouts for Beginners," the perfect starting point for those new to fitness or returning after a hiatus. This chapter will guide you through introductory sessions designed to ease you into a regular exercise routine while building confidence and strength. By following these beginner-friendly workouts, you'll lay a solid foundation that prepares you for the more advanced routines covered in Part 2. Combining the insights from Chapter 8, we ensure that even as a beginner, you can mix and balance your workouts effectively.

Starting Slow: Introductory Sessions

Embarking on a fitness journey can be daunting, but starting slow with well-structured introductory sessions can make the process enjoyable and sustainable. These sessions focus on simple, low-impact exercises that build a base level of fitness without overwhelming you.

Benefits of Starting Slow:

- **Reduces Risk of Injury:** Gradually increasing intensity helps your body adapt, reducing the risk of injury.
- **Builds Habits:** Starting slow allows you to develop a consistent exercise habit without feeling burned out.
- **Boosts Confidence:** Successfully completing beginner workouts boosts your confidence and motivation to

continue.

Sample Introductory Session:

1. **Warm-Up:** 5 minutes of gentle walking or marching in place.

2. **Workout:**
   - **Bodyweight Squats**: 10 reps
   - **Modified Push-Ups**: 10 reps
   - **Standing Marches**: 1 minute
   - **Seated Rows with Resistance Band**: 10 reps
   - **Standing Calf Raises**: 10 reps

3. **Repeat:** Perform the circuit 2 times with a short rest between sets.

4. **Cool Down:** 5 minutes of stretching, focusing on major muscle groups.

Introductory Tips:

- Focus on form over speed or intensity to build a solid foundation.
- Take breaks as needed and listen to your body to avoid overexertion.
- Celebrate small victories and progress, no matter how incremental.

Building Confidence and Strength

As you become more comfortable with your introductory sessions, it's time to build confidence and strength. These workouts gradually increase in intensity and complexity, helping you develop a stronger, more resilient body.

Benefits of Building Confidence and Strength:

- **Progressive Improvement:** Gradually challenging your body helps you see and feel progress, boosting motivation.
- **Foundation for Advanced Workouts:** Building strength

and confidence prepares you for more complex routines.

- **Enhanced Well-Being:** Physical strength translates to improved mental and emotional well-being, fostering a positive outlook.

Sample Confidence-Building Workout:

1. **Warm-Up:** 5 minutes of light cardio, such as brisk walking or stationary cycling.

2. **Workout:**
   - **Lunges**: 10 reps per leg
   - **Plank (Knees Down)**: Hold for 20 seconds
   - **Dumbbell Chest Press**: 10 reps
   - **Bent-Over Dumbbell Rows**: 10 reps per side
   - **Side Leg Lifts**: 10 reps per leg

3. **Repeat:** Perform the circuit 3 times, with rest as needed between sets.

4. **Cool Down:** 5 minutes of stretching, focusing on flexibility and muscle relaxation.

Building Tips:

- Increase the weight or repetitions gradually as your strength improves.

- Incorporate a mix of compound and isolation exercises to target different muscle groups.

- Maintain a positive mindset, focusing on progress rather than perfection.

By starting slow and progressively building strength and confidence, you'll establish a solid fitness foundation that supports more advanced workouts. These beginner routines align with the principles of combining and balancing workouts from Chapter 8, ensuring a holistic approach to your fitness journey.

CHAPTER 10: ADVANCED CHALLENGES

Welcome to "Advanced Challenges," the pinnacle of the "Fit in a Flash" program designed for those ready to push their limits and achieve peak fitness. This chapter features high-intensity sessions and advanced strength circuits that will challenge your body and elevate your fitness level. Building on the foundation established in Chapter 9's beginner workouts, these advanced routines are designed to maximize results and keep you motivated with new and exciting challenges.

Pushing Limits: High-Intensity Sessions

High-intensity sessions are perfect for those looking to take their fitness to the next level. These workouts combine explosive movements with minimal rest periods to maximize calorie burn, increase endurance, and build muscle strength.

Benefits of High-Intensity Sessions:

- **Maximal Calorie Burn:** Burn more calories in a shorter amount of time compared to traditional workouts.
- **Improved Endurance:** High-intensity exercises boost cardiovascular fitness and stamina.
- **Increased Metabolic Rate:** Continue burning calories even after the workout is done due to the afterburn effect.

Sample High-Intensity Session:

1. **Warm-Up**: 5 minutes of dynamic stretching and light cardio.
2. **Workout:**
   - **Burpees**: 1 minute
   - **Kettlebell Swings**: 1 minute
   - **Jump Squats**: 1 minute
   - **Mountain Climbers**: 1 minute
   - **High Knees**: 1 minute
3. **Rest:** 1 minute between circuits.
4. **Repeat:** Perform the circuit 4 times.
5. **Cool Down:** 5 minutes of static stretching, focusing on the muscles used.

High-Intensity Tips:

- Maintain proper form to avoid injury, even when working at high speeds.
- Listen to your body and adjust the intensity if needed.
- Stay hydrated and ensure you are properly fueled for these demanding workouts.

Advanced Strength Circuits

Advanced strength circuits are designed to build muscle, increase strength, and enhance overall physical performance. These circuits involve compound movements that target multiple muscle groups, ensuring a comprehensive workout.

Benefits of Advanced Strength Circuits:

- **Muscle Growth:** Stimulate muscle hypertrophy through challenging and varied exercises.
- **Functional Strength:** Improve strength that translates into better performance in everyday activities.
- **Balanced Development:** Target multiple muscle groups for well-rounded fitness.

Sample Advanced Strength Circuit:

1. **Warm-Up:** 5 minutes of light cardio and mobility exercises.
2. **Workout:**
   - **Deadlifts**: 12 reps
   - **Pull-Ups**: 10 reps
   - **Barbell Squats**: 12 reps
   - **Overhead Press**: 10 reps
   - **Dumbbell Bench Press**: 12 reps
3. **Rest:** 1-2 minutes between sets.
4. **Repeat:** Perform the circuit 3 times.
5. **Cool Down:** 5 minutes of stretching, focusing on flexibility and recovery.

Advanced Strength Tips:

- Use weights that challenge you but allow you to maintain proper form.
- Increase the weight progressively as your strength improves.
- Focus on compound movements that engage multiple muscle groups for maximum efficiency.

By incorporating these high-intensity sessions and advanced strength circuits into your routine, you'll achieve a new level of fitness and strength. These advanced workouts build on the basics from Chapter 9, ensuring you have the foundation needed to tackle more challenging routines.

CHAPTER 11: WORKOUTS FOR SPECIFIC GOALS

Welcome to "Workouts for Specific Goals," a chapter tailored to help you achieve your unique fitness aspirations. Whether you're aiming for weight loss, muscle toning, or stress relief and mental clarity, this chapter provides specialized workouts designed to meet your needs. Building on the advanced challenges from Chapter 10, these targeted routines ensure you can focus on your personal fitness goals while continuing to push your limits.

Weight Loss

If weight loss is your primary goal, incorporating high-intensity cardio with strength training is key. These workouts are designed to maximize calorie burn, boost your metabolism, and enhance fat loss.

Benefits of Weight Loss Workouts:

- **Calorie Burn:** Efficiently burn calories through high-intensity exercises.
- **Fat Reduction:** Target stored body fat with metabolic-boosting routines.
- **Improved Health:** Achieve a healthier body weight, reducing the risk of chronic diseases.

Sample Weight Loss Workout:

1. **Warm-Up:** 5 minutes of brisk walking or jogging.
2. **Workout:**

- **Jump Rope:** 2 minutes
- **Burpees:** 1 minute
- **Squat Jumps:** 1 minute
- **Mountain Climbers:** 1 minute
- **Dumbbell Thrusters:** 1 minute

3. **Rest:** 1 minute between sets.
4. **Repeat:** Perform the circuit 3-4 times.
5. **Cool Down:** 5 minutes of stretching, focusing on major muscle groups.

Weight Loss Tips:

- Keep the intensity high to maximize calorie expenditure.
- Combine these workouts with a balanced, calorie-controlled diet for best results.
- Track your progress and adjust your routine as needed to continue seeing results.

Muscle Toning

For those focused on muscle toning, the goal is to define and sculpt your muscles without necessarily increasing bulk. These workouts emphasize high repetitions with moderate weights and incorporate bodyweight exercises to enhance muscle definition.

Benefits of Muscle Toning Workouts:

- **Muscle Definition:** Achieve a lean, sculpted appearance.
- **Functional Strength:** Improve muscle endurance and functionality.
- **Body Composition:** Enhance overall body composition by increasing lean muscle mass.

Sample Muscle Toning Workout:

1. **Warm-Up:** 5 minutes of light cardio and dynamic stretches.
2. **Workout:**

- **Push-Ups:** 15 reps
- **Dumbbell Lateral Raises:** 15 reps
- **Bodyweight Lunges:** 15 reps per leg
- **Plank with Shoulder Taps:** 15 reps per side
- **Russian Twists:** 20 reps per side

3. **Rest:** 1 minute between sets.

4. **Repeat:** Perform the circuit 3 times.

5. **Cool Down:** 5 minutes of stretching, focusing on flexibility and muscle recovery.

Muscle Toning Tips:

- Focus on form and control to target specific muscle groups effectively.
- Use weights that allow you to complete the reps with good form but feel challenging by the last few reps.
- Incorporate a mix of bodyweight and resistance exercises for balanced muscle development.

Stress Relief and Mental Clarity

Workouts that focus on stress relief and mental clarity are essential for overall well-being. These routines combine gentle movements, mindfulness, and stretching to reduce stress and enhance mental clarity.

Benefits of Stress Relief Workouts:

- **Reduced Stress:** Lower cortisol levels and promote relaxation.
- **Improved Mental Clarity:** Enhance focus and mental sharpness.
- **Holistic Health:** Support mental and emotional well-being alongside physical health.

Sample Stress Relief Workout:

1. **Warm-Up:** 5 minutes of deep breathing and gentle stretching.

2. **Workout:**
   - **Child's Pose:** 2 minutes
   - **Cat-Cow Stretch:** 1 minute
   - **Downward Dog:** 1 minute
   - **Seated Forward Bend:** 2 minutes
   - **Legs-Up-the-Wall Pose:** 5 minutes
3. **Cool Down:** 5 minutes of deep breathing and relaxation in Corpse Pose (Savasana).

Stress Relief Tips:

- Focus on your breath and move slowly through each pose to maximize relaxation.
- Incorporate these workouts into your routine regularly to manage stress effectively.
- Pair physical activity with other stress-relief practices such as meditation or journaling.

By targeting specific fitness goals with these tailored workouts, you can achieve the results you desire while maintaining a balanced and enjoyable exercise routine. These specialized workouts complement the advanced challenges from Chapter 10, ensuring you have a comprehensive toolkit to reach your fitness aspirations.

Part 4: Lifestyle Integration

CHAPTER 12: HEALTHY EATING ON A TIGHT SCHEDULE

Nutrition Basics for Busy Lives

In the hustle and bustle of everyday life, maintaining a nutritious diet can seem daunting. However, understanding the basics of nutrition and how to apply them efficiently can make a world of difference. Proper nutrition not only fuels your workouts but also enhances overall health, boosts energy levels, and aids in recovery.

Key Principles:

1. **Balanced Macronutrients**: Aim for a balance of proteins, carbohydrates, and healthy fats. Proteins are essential for muscle repair and growth, carbohydrates provide energy, and fats support cell function and hormone production.

2. **Micronutrient Essentials**: Ensure you're getting enough vitamins and minerals through a varied diet rich in fruits, vegetables, lean proteins, and whole grains.

3. **Hydration**: Staying hydrated is crucial. Aim to drink at least eight glasses of water a day, more if you're active. Water helps with digestion, nutrient transport, and temperature regulation.

4. **Meal Timing**: Eating small, balanced meals throughout the day can help maintain energy levels and prevent overeating. Aim for three main meals and two snacks.

By focusing on these nutrition basics, you can create a solid foundation for a healthy diet that supports your fitness goals, even with a busy schedule.

Quick and Healthy Meal Ideas

Eating healthy doesn't have to be time-consuming. With a little planning and some smart choices, you can whip up nutritious meals in no time. Here are some quick and healthy meal ideas that fit perfectly into a hectic lifestyle:

Breakfast:

1. **Overnight Oats**: Combine oats, milk (or a dairy-free alternative), chia seeds, and your favorite fruits in a jar. Let it sit in the fridge overnight, and you'll have a nutritious breakfast ready to go.

2. **Smoothie Packs**: Pre-pack smoothie ingredients (fruits, spinach, protein powder) in freezer bags. In the morning, just blend with some liquid for a quick, nutrient-dense meal.

Lunch:

1. **Mason Jar Salads**: Layer your favorite salad ingredients in a mason jar (dressing at the bottom, sturdy veggies and proteins in the middle, and greens on top). Shake and eat when ready.

2. **Wraps and Sandwiches**: Use whole grain wraps or bread, lean proteins (chicken, turkey, tofu), and plenty of veggies. Add hummus or avocado for extra flavor and nutrients.

Dinner:

1. **One-Pan Meals**: Toss protein (chicken, fish, tofu), veggies, and some olive oil and spices onto a baking sheet. Roast in the oven for a simple, balanced dinner.

2. **Stir-Fries**: Quickly cook protein and vegetables in a hot pan with a bit of oil and your favorite sauce. Serve over brown rice or quinoa.

Snacks:

1. <u>**Energy Bites**: Combine oats, nut butter, honey, and mix-ins like chocolate chips or dried fruit. Roll into balls and refrigerate.</u>

2. <u>**Veggie Sticks and Hummus**: Pre-cut vegetables like carrots, celery, and bell peppers, and pair with store-bought or homemade hummus.</u>

Meal Prep Tips:

- <u>**Plan Ahead**: Dedicate a couple of hours each week to meal prep. Prepare ingredients in bulk, like chopping vegetables or cooking grains, to save time during the week.</u>

- <u>**Batch Cooking**: Make large batches of soups, stews, or casseroles that can be portioned out and frozen for future meals.</u>

- <u>**Smart Storage**: Invest in good-quality, reusable containers to keep your prepped food fresh and portable.</u>

By integrating these quick and healthy meal ideas into your routine, you can maintain a nutritious diet that complements your fitness efforts, even with a packed schedule. Remember, eating well is just as important as exercising when it comes to achieving your health and fitness goals. Let "Fit in a Flash" guide you not only in your workouts but also in making smart, time-efficient nutritional choices that support a balanced, healthy lifestyle.

PART 4: LIFESTYLE INTEGRATION

CHAPTER 13: TRACKING PROGRESS AND STAYING MOTIVATED

Keeping track of your fitness journey and staying motivated are essential components of achieving lasting success. In "Fit in a Flash: 30-Minute Workouts for Busy Lives," we provide you with effective tools and strategies to ensure you remain committed and inspired. This chapter explores the benefits of using fitness journals and apps, and the importance of celebrating milestones along the way.

Using Fitness Journals and Apps

Fitness Journals:

- **The Power of Writing**: Recording your workouts, meals, and feelings in a fitness journal can significantly boost your motivation and accountability. It helps you see patterns, track progress, and stay focused on your goals.

- **What to Track**: Include details like the type and duration of your workouts, the intensity level, any physical or emotional changes, and nutritional intake. Also, jot down reflections on what worked well and areas for improvement.

- **Setting Goals**: Use your journal to set short-term and long-term goals. Breaking down larger objectives into manageable tasks can make the journey less overwhelming and more achievable.

- **Visualization**: Seeing your progress on paper can be incredibly motivating. It provides a tangible record of your hard work and dedication.

Fitness Apps:

- **Convenience at Your Fingertips**: Fitness apps offer an easy and efficient way to monitor your progress. Many apps come with features like workout tracking, meal planning, and progress analytics.

- **Top Picks**: Consider using popular apps like MyFitnessPal, Strava, or Fitbit, which offer comprehensive tracking and motivational tools.

- **Customizable Workouts**: Many apps provide personalized workout plans based on your fitness level and goals. They also offer video tutorials to ensure proper form and technique.

- **Community Support**: Joining app-based communities can provide additional motivation. Sharing achievements and challenges with others can create a supportive and encouraging environment.

Celebrating Milestones

Recognizing and celebrating your achievements, no matter how small, is crucial for maintaining motivation and a positive mindset. Here's how you can effectively celebrate your milestones:

Setting Milestones:

- **Short-Term Milestones**: Set achievable goals like completing a certain number of workouts per week or increasing the intensity of your exercises. These small wins build confidence and keep you moving forward.

- **Long-Term Milestones**: Establish larger goals such as reaching a specific weight, completing a fitness challenge, or running a race. These long-term milestones provide a sense of purpose and direction.

Ways to Celebrate:

- **Reward Yourself**: Treat yourself to something special when you hit a milestone. This could be new workout gear, a relaxing spa day, or a favorite healthy treat. Rewards provide positive reinforcement and make the journey enjoyable.

- **Share Your Success**: Celebrate with friends, family, or your fitness community. Sharing your achievements can boost your motivation and inspire others.

- **Reflect on Your Journey**: Take time to reflect on how far you've come. Revisit your fitness journal or app entries to see the progress you've made. This reflection can reignite your passion and commitment.

Visual Reminders:

- **Progress Photos**: Take regular progress photos to visually track your transformation. Comparing photos over time can be incredibly motivating.

- **Achievement Boards**: Create a board where you can display your goals and milestones. Adding visual elements like stickers or photos can make this a fun and inspiring tool.

By using fitness journals and apps to track your progress and celebrating milestones along the way, you stay engaged and motivated in your fitness journey. "Fit in a Flash: 30-Minute Workouts for Busy Lives" isn't just about quick workouts—it's about integrating a healthy, balanced lifestyle that you can maintain and enjoy. Embrace these tools and strategies to stay on track and make your fitness goals a reality.

CHAPTER 14: BALANCING FITNESS WITH DAILY LIFE

Maintaining a consistent fitness routine while managing a busy schedule can be challenging, but it's entirely possible with the right strategies. In "Fit in a Flash: 30-Minute Workouts for Busy Lives," we've covered effective workout routines, healthy eating habits, and tracking progress. Now, let's explore how to seamlessly integrate fitness into your daily life and stay active beyond traditional workouts.

Integrating Workouts into Your Routine

Finding time for exercise in a hectic schedule requires creativity and planning. Here are some tips to help you make fitness a natural part of your day:

Morning Workouts:

- **Start Your Day Right**: Morning workouts can jumpstart your metabolism and boost your energy levels for the day ahead. Set your alarm 30 minutes earlier and use that time for a quick, effective workout from "Fit in a Flash."

- **Consistency is Key**: Establish a morning routine that includes exercise. Over time, it will become a habit, making it easier to stick with.

Lunch Break Workouts:

- **Utilize Breaks**: If mornings are too hectic, use your

lunch break for a workout. A 30-minute session can refresh your mind and increase afternoon productivity.

- **Convenience Matters**: Keep workout clothes and a water bottle at your desk. Choose exercises that don't require much equipment, like bodyweight routines or resistance band exercises.

Evening Workouts:

- **Wind Down with Exercise**: If evenings are more convenient, incorporate a workout into your wind-down routine. It can help relieve stress accumulated throughout the day.

- **Family Involvement**: Turn your workout into family time. Engage in activities everyone can enjoy, such as a family walk or a mini home workout session.

Micro Workouts:

- **Short Bursts**: When time is extremely limited, break your workout into smaller segments throughout the day. Even 10-minute bursts of exercise can add up to significant health benefits.

- **Flexibility**: Incorporate exercises during TV commercials, while waiting for meals to cook, or during any idle moments.

Staying Active Outside the Gym

Fitness isn't confined to the gym. Staying active throughout the day can enhance your overall health and complement your workout routine. Here are ways to keep moving:

Active Commuting:

- **Walk or Bike**: If possible, walk or bike to work instead of driving. This integrates physical activity into your daily routine effortlessly.

- **Public Transport**: If you use public transport, try getting off a stop early and walking the rest of the way.

Desk Exercises:

- **Stretch Breaks**: Incorporate short stretch breaks throughout your workday to prevent stiffness and improve circulation.
- **Chair Exercises**: Perform simple exercises like seated leg lifts or desk push-ups to stay active while working.

Household Chores:

- **Active Cleaning**: Turn cleaning into a workout. Vacuuming, sweeping, and gardening can burn significant calories and keep you moving.
- **DIY Projects**: Engage in home improvement tasks that require physical effort, such as painting or rearranging furniture.

Outdoor Activities:

- **Nature Walks**: Spend time outdoors with activities like hiking, walking, or running in a local park. Fresh air and nature can boost your mood and energy.
- **Playtime**: Engage in physical play with your children or pets. Activities like playing catch, frisbee, or a game of tag can be fun and active.

Social Activities:

- **Group Sports**: Join a local sports league or participate in group fitness classes. This adds a social element to your fitness routine, making it more enjoyable.
- **Fitness Meetups**: Participate in community fitness events or meetups. This can be a great way to stay motivated and meet like-minded individuals.

Balancing fitness with daily life requires flexibility and creativity. By integrating workouts into your routine and finding ways to stay active throughout the day, you can achieve a healthy, balanced lifestyle without feeling overwhelmed. Remember, every bit of activity counts, and consistency is key. Embrace these strategies to make fitness a seamless part of your busy life and enjoy the transformative benefits it brings.

CONCLUSION: THE JOURNEY AHEAD

As you reach the end of "Fit in a Flash: 30-Minute Workouts for Busy Lives," it's time to reflect on your accomplishments and look forward to the journey ahead. Embracing fitness as a lifelong commitment requires maintaining momentum and adapting to the inevitable changes in your life. This concluding chapter offers guidance on how to stay motivated and flexible, ensuring your fitness journey continues to thrive.

Maintaining Momentum

Consistency is the cornerstone of any successful fitness regimen. Maintaining the momentum you've built with your 30-minute workouts will help you continue reaping the benefits of your hard work.

Stay Engaged:

- **Variety is Key**: Keep your workouts interesting by regularly mixing up your routine. Try new exercises, different workout styles, or varying the intensity to prevent boredom and keep your body challenged.
- **Set New Goals**: As you achieve your initial goals, set new ones to strive for. Whether it's running a longer distance, lifting heavier weights, or mastering a new skill, having something to work towards keeps you motivated.

Stay Connected:

- **Fitness Community**: Engage with a fitness community,

either online or in-person. Sharing your journey with others can provide support, accountability, and inspiration.

- **Track Progress**: Continue using fitness journals or apps to track your progress. Seeing your achievements over time can boost your motivation and help you stay on course.

Stay Positive:

- **Celebrate Wins**: Regularly acknowledge and celebrate your accomplishments, no matter how small. Positive reinforcement encourages a healthy mindset and keeps you motivated.

- **Focus on the Benefits**: Remind yourself of the numerous benefits you've experienced from staying active—improved energy, better mood, enhanced strength, and overall well-being.

Adapting as Your Life Changes

Life is full of changes, and your fitness routine should adapt accordingly. Whether you're facing a new job, family obligations, or health changes, flexibility is essential to maintaining your fitness journey.

Life Transitions:

- **New Routines**: Major life changes, like a new job or moving to a new city, can disrupt your routine. Plan ahead and create new workout schedules that fit your current lifestyle.

- **Stay Flexible**: Be open to adjusting your fitness goals and routines. If you can't fit in a full workout, shorter, high-intensity sessions or micro workouts can keep you on track.

Family and Social Life:

- **Include Loved Ones**: Involve your family and friends in your fitness activities. Family walks, group sports, or workout challenges can make staying active a fun, shared experience.

- **Time Management**: Efficiently manage your time to balance fitness with family and social commitments. Prioritize activities that contribute to your overall well-being.

Health Considerations:

- **Listen to Your Body**: As you age or face health issues, it's important to listen to your body. Modify workouts to suit your current fitness level and consult with healthcare professionals if needed.

- **Adapt Workouts**: Adjust the intensity and type of exercises to match your physical capabilities. Focus on low-impact activities like swimming, yoga, or walking if high-intensity workouts become challenging.

Mindset Shifts:

- **Embrace Change**: View changes as opportunities to grow and evolve your fitness journey. Adaptability is a strength that can help you stay active and healthy despite life's ups and downs.

- **Continuous Learning**: Stay informed about new fitness trends, exercises, and health tips. Continual learning keeps your fitness routine fresh and aligned with your evolving goals.

Your journey with "Fit in a Flash: 30-Minute Workouts for Busy Lives" is just the beginning. By maintaining momentum and adapting to life's changes, you'll ensure that fitness remains an integral and enjoyable part of your life. Embrace the journey ahead with confidence, flexibility, and a positive mindset. Here's to a healthier, happier, and more active you!

RESOURCES AND FURTHER READING

As you conclude your journey through "Fit in a Flash: 30-Minute Workouts for Busy Lives," equipping yourself with additional resources and knowledge can further enhance your fitness journey. This section provides recommendations for helpful apps and tools, as well as further reading on fitness and health to support your continued growth and success.

Recommended Apps and Tools

In the digital age, a variety of apps and tools can streamline your fitness routine, keep you motivated, and help you track your progress effectively. Here are some top recommendations to consider:

Fitness Tracking Apps:

- **MyFitnessPal**: A comprehensive app for tracking your diet and exercise. It features a vast food database, barcode scanning, and personalized goal setting.

- **Strava**: Ideal for runners and cyclists, Strava tracks your workouts via GPS, provides performance analytics, and offers a social community for added motivation.

- **Fitbit**: Sync your Fitbit device with this app to monitor your steps, heart rate, sleep patterns, and more. It's perfect for those looking to get detailed insights into their daily activity.

Workout Apps:

- **Nike Training Club**: Offers a variety of workouts

designed by professional trainers, ranging from strength and endurance to mobility and yoga.

- **7 Minute Workout**: For those who are extremely pressed for time, this app offers quick, high-intensity workouts that can be done anywhere.
- **Centr**: Created by Chris Hemsworth, this app provides workouts, meal plans, and mindfulness exercises tailored to your fitness level and goals.

Nutrition Apps:

- **Yummly**: Personalized recipe recommendations based on your dietary preferences and restrictions. It also features shopping list creation and meal planning.
- **Lose It!**: A user-friendly app for calorie counting and weight loss. It helps you set goals, track food intake, and monitor your progress.

Mindfulness and Recovery Apps:

- **Headspace**: Offers guided meditation and mindfulness exercises to help reduce stress and improve mental well-being.
- **Calm**: Focuses on sleep, meditation, and relaxation, providing tools to enhance your overall mental health.

Further Reading on Fitness and Health

Continual learning is crucial for staying informed and motivated on your fitness journey. Here are some highly recommended books and resources to deepen your understanding of fitness and health:

Fitness and Exercise:

- **"The New Rules of Lifting for Women" by Lou Schuler and Alwyn Cosgrove**: A comprehensive guide to strength training designed specifically for women.
- **"Body by Science" by John R. Little and Doug McGuff**: Explores the science behind high-intensity training and

its benefits for muscle growth and fat loss.

- **"Starting Strength: Basic Barbell Training" by Mark Rippetoe**: A detailed guide to barbell training, perfect for those looking to improve their strength and technique.

Nutrition and Diet:

- **"The Whole30: The 30-Day Guide to Total Health and Food Freedom" by Melissa Hartwig Urban and Dallas Hartwig**: A guide to resetting your eating habits with a 30-day nutrition plan.

- **"In Defense of Food: An Eater's Manifesto" by Michael Pollan**: Offers insights into making healthier food choices and understanding modern dietary issues.

- **"The Plant Paradox: The Hidden Dangers in 'Healthy' Foods That Cause Disease and Weight Gain" by Dr. Steven R. Gundry**: Discusses the potential health impacts of certain plant-based foods and offers dietary recommendations.

Mindfulness and Well-being:

- **"The Power of Now: A Guide to Spiritual Enlightenment" by Eckhart Tolle**: Focuses on the importance of living in the present moment for mental clarity and peace.

- **"Why We Sleep: Unlocking the Power of Sleep and Dreams" by Matthew Walker**: Explores the critical role of sleep in our overall health and offers practical tips for improving sleep quality.

General Health:

- **"How Not to Die: Discover the Foods Scientifically Proven to Prevent and Reverse Disease" by Dr. Michael Greger**: Provides evidence-based dietary advice for preventing common diseases.

- **"Spark: The Revolutionary New Science of Exercise and the Brain" by John J. Ratey**: Examines the profound

<u>impact of physical exercise on brain health and cognitive function.</u>

By utilizing these recommended apps and tools, and diving into further reading, you'll be well-equipped to continue your fitness journey with a wealth of knowledge and resources at your fingertips. Keep exploring, learning, and growing as you strive for a healthier, more active life.